INSULIN RESISTANCE DIET

MAIN COURSE - 60+ Breakfast, Lunch, Dinner and Dessert Recipes for Insulin Resistance Diet

TABLE OF CONTENTS

purposes solely, and is universal as so. The presentation of the information is without contract or any type of guarantee assurance.

The trademarks that are used are without any consent, and the publication of the trademark is without permission or backing by the trademark owner. All trademarks and brands within this book are for clarifying purposes only and are the owned by the owners themselves, not affiliated with this document.

Introduction

Insulin Resistance recipes for personal enjoyment but also for family enjoyment. You will love them for sure for how easy it is to prepare them.

BLUEBERRY PANCAKES

Serves: *4*
Prep Time: *10* Minutes

Cook Time: *20* Minutes

Total Time: *30* Minutes

INGREDIENTS

- 1 cup whole wheat flour
- ¼ tsp baking soda
- ¼ tsp baking powder
- 1 cup blueberries
- 2 eggs
- 1 cup milk

DIRECTIONS

1. In a bowl combine all ingredients together and mix well
2. In a skillet heat olive oil

3. Pour ¼ of the batter and cook each pancake for 1-2 minutes per side

4. When ready remove from heat and serve

PEACH PANCAKES

Serves: *4*

Prep Time: *10*   Minutes

Cook Time: *30*   Minutes

Total Time: *40*   Minutes

INGREDIENTS

- 1 cup whole wheat flour
- ¼ tsp baking soda
- ¼ tsp baking powder
- 1 cup mashed peaches
- 2 eggs
- 1 cup milk

DIRECTIONS

1. In a bowl combine all ingredients together and mix well

2. In a skillet heat olive oil

3. Pour ¼ of the batter and cook each pancake for 1-2 minutes per side

4. When ready remove from heat and serve

Serves: *4*

Prep Time: *10* Minutes

Cook Time: *20* Minutes

Total Time: *30* Minutes

INGREDIENTS

- 1 cup whole wheat flour
- ¼ tsp baking soda
- ¼ tsp baking powder
- 1 cup mashed banana
- 2 eggs
- 1 cup milk

DIRECTIONS

1. In a bowl combine all ingredients together and mix well
2. In a skillet heat olive oil
3. Pour ¼ of the batter and cook each pancake for 1-2 minutes per side

4. When ready remove from heat and serve

12

PLUMS PANCAKES

Serves: *4*
Prep Time: *10*   Minutes

Cook Time: *20*   Minutes

Total Time: *30*   Minutes

INGREDIENTS

- 1 cup whole wheat flour
- ¼ tsp baking soda
- ¼ tsp baking powder
- 1 cup mashed plums
- 2 eggs
- 1 cup milk

DIRECTIONS

1. In a bowl combine all ingredients together and mix well

2. In a skillet heat olive oil

3. Pour ¼ of the batter and cook each pancake for 1-2 minutes per side

4. When ready remove from heat and serve

14

Serves: **4**

Prep Time: **10** Minutes

Cook Time: **30** Minutes

Total Time: **40** Minutes

INGREDIENTS

- 1 cup whole wheat flour
- ¼ tsp baking soda
- ¼ tsp baking powder
- 2 eggs
- 1 cup milk

DIRECTIONS

1. In a bowl combine all ingredients together and mix well
2. In a skillet heat olive oil
3. Pour ¼ of the batter and cook each pancake for 1-2 minutes per side
4. When ready remove from heat and serve

Serves: *8-12*
Prep Time: *10*   Minutes

Cook Time: *20*   Minutes

Total Time: *30*   Minutes

INGREDIENTS

- 2 eggs
- 1 tablespoon olive oil
- 1 cup milk
- 2 cups whole wheat flour
- 1 tsp baking soda
- ¼ tsp baking soda
- 1 tsp ginger
- 1 tsp cinnamon
- ¼ cup molasses

DIRECTIONS

1. In a bowl combine all dry ingredients
2. In another bowl combine all dry ingredients

3. Combine wet and dry ingredients together

4. Fold in ginger and mix well

5. Pour mixture into 8-12 prepared muffin cups, fill 2/3 of the cups

6. Bake for 18-20 minutes at 375 F

7. When ready remove from the oven and serve

KIWI MUFFINS

Serves: *8-12*
Prep Time: *10*   Minutes

Cook Time: *20*   Minutes

Total Time: *30*   Minutes

INGREDIENTS

- 2 eggs
- 1 tablespoon olive oil
- 1 cup milk
- 2 cups whole wheat flour
- 1 tsp baking soda
- ¼ tsp baking soda
- 1 tsp cinnamon
- 1 cup mashed kiwi

DIRECTIONS

1. In a bowl combine all dry ingredients
2. In another bowl combine all dry ingredients
3. Combine wet and dry ingredients together

4. Pour mixture into 8-12 prepared muffin cups, fill 2/3 of the cups

5. Bake for 18-20 minutes at 375 F

6. When ready remove from the oven and serve

Serves:	**8-12**	
Prep Time:	**10**	Minutes
Cook Time:	**20**	Minutes
Total Time:	**30**	Minutes

INGREDIENTS

- 2 eggs
- 1 tablespoon olive oil
- 1 cup milk
- 2 cups whole wheat flour
- 1 tsp baking soda
- ¼ tsp baking soda
- 1 tsp cinnamon
- 1 cup blueberries

DIRECTIONS

1. In a bowl combine all dry ingredients
2. In another bowl combine all dry ingredients
3. Combine wet and dry ingredients together

4. Pour mixture into 8-12 prepared muffin cups, fill
    2/3 of the cups

5. Bake for 18-20 minutes at 375 F

6. When ready remove from the oven and serve

Serves:	*8-12*	
Prep Time:	*10*	Minutes
Cook Time:	*20*	Minutes
Total Time:	*30*	Minutes

INGREDIENTS

- 2 eggs
- 1 tablespoon olive oil
- 1 cup milk
- 2 cups whole wheat flour
- 1 tsp baking soda
- ¼ tsp baking soda
- 1 tsp cinnamon
- 1 cup mashed plums

DIRECTIONS

1. In a bowl combine all dry ingredients
2. In another bowl combine all dry ingredients
3. Combine wet and dry ingredients together

4. Pour mixture into 8-12 prepared muffin cups, fill 2/3 of the cups

5. Bake for 18-20 minutes at 375 F

6. When ready remove from the oven and serve

Serves: **8-12**

Prep Time: **10** Minutes

Cook Time: **20** Minutes

Total Time: **30** Minutes

INGREDIENTS

- 2 eggs
- 1 tablespoon olive oil
- 1 cup milk
- 2 cups whole wheat flour
- 1 tsp baking soda
- ¼ tsp baking soda
- 1 tsp cinnamon
- 1 cup chocolate chips

DIRECTIONS

1. In a bowl combine all dry ingredients
2. In another bowl combine all dry ingredients
3. Combine wet and dry ingredients together

4. Fold in chocolate chips and mix well

5. Pour mixture into 8-12 prepared muffin cups, fill
    2/3 of the cups

6. Bake for 18-20 minutes at 375 F

7. When ready remove from the oven and serve

Serves:	*8-12*
Prep Time:	*10* Minutes
Cook Time:	*20* Minutes
Total Time:	*30* Minutes

INGREDIENTS

- 2 eggs
- 1 tablespoon olive oil
- 1 cup milk
- 2 cups whole wheat flour
- 1 tsp baking soda
- 1 cup mashed prunes
- ¼ tsp baking soda
- 1 tsp cinnamon
- 1 cup mashed prunes

DIRECTIONS

1. In a bowl combine all dry ingredients
2. In another bowl combine all dry ingredients

3. Combine wet and dry ingredients together

4. Pour mixture into 8-12 prepared muffin cups, fill
    2/3 of the cups

5. Bake for 18-20 minutes at 375 F

6. When ready remove from the oven and serve

OLIVE OMELETTE

Serves: *1*
Prep Time: *5*   Minutes

Cook Time: *10*   Minutes

Total Time: *15*   Minutes

INGREDIENTS

- **2 eggs**
- **¼ tsp salt**
- **¼ tsp black pepper**
- **1 tablespoon olive oil**
- **¼ cup cheese**
- **½ cup olives**
- **¼ tsp basil**

DIRECTIONS

1. **In a bowl combine all ingredients together and mix well**
2. **In a skillet heat olive oil and pour the egg mixture**

3. Cook for 1-2 minutes per side

4. When ready remove omelette from the skillet and
    serve

ZUCCHINI OMELETTE

Serves: *1*

Prep Time: *5* Minutes

Cook Time: *10* Minutes

Total Time: *15* Minutes

INGREDIENTS

- **2 eggs**
- **¼ tsp salt**
- **¼ tsp black pepper**
- **1 tablespoon olive oil**
- **¼ cup cheese**
- **¼ tsp basil**
- **1 cup zucchini**

DIRECTIONS

1. **In a bowl combine all ingredients together and mix well**
2. **In a skillet heat olive oil and pour the egg mixture**

3. Cook for 1-2 minutes per side

4. When ready remove omelette from the skillet and
   serve

BASIL OMELETTE

Serves: **1**

Prep Time: **5** Minutes

Cook Time: **10** Minutes

Total Time: **15** Minutes

INGREDIENTS

- **2 eggs**
- **¼ tsp salt**
- **¼ tsp black pepper**
- **1 tablespoon olive oil**
- **¼ cup cheese**
- **¼ tsp basil**
- **1 cup red onion**

DIRECTIONS

1. **In a bowl combine all ingredients together and mix well**

2. **In a skillet heat olive oil and pour the egg mixture**

3. Cook for 1-2 minutes per side

4. When ready remove omelette from the skillet and serve

MUSHROOM OMELETTE

Serves: *1*
Prep Time: *5* Minutes

Cook Time: *10* Minutes

Total Time: *15* Minutes

INGREDIENTS

- 2 eggs
- ¼ tsp salt
- ¼ tsp black pepper
- 1 tablespoon olive oil
- ¼ cup cheese
- ¼ tsp basil
- 1 cup mushrooms

DIRECTIONS

1. In a bowl combine all ingredients together and mix well
2. In a skillet heat olive oil and pour the egg mixture

3. Cook for 1-2 minutes per side

4. When ready remove omelette from the skillet and
    serve

Serves: *1*

Prep Time: *5*   Minutes

Cook Time: *10*   Minutes

Total Time: *15*   Minutes

INGREDIENTS

- 2 eggs
- ¼ tsp salt
- ¼ tsp black pepper
- 1 tablespoon olive oil
- ¼ cup cheese
- ¼ tsp basil
- 1 cup tomatoes

DIRECTIONS

1. In a bowl combine all ingredients together and mix well

2. In a skillet heat olive oil and pour the egg mixture

3. Cook for 1-2 minutes per side

4. When ready remove omelette from the skillet and
    serve

Serves: 2

Prep Time: 5   Minutes

Cook Time: *10*   Minutes

Total Time: *15*   Minutes

INGREDIENTS

- 2 cups oats
- 1 cup strawberries
- 1 tablespoon chia seeds
- 1 banana
- 2 cups almond milk
- 1 tablespoon maple syrup

DIRECTIONS

1. Mash banana and strawberries together, set aside
2. In a saucepan add the rest of the ingredients and bring to a boil
3. Reduce heat and cook for 4-5 minutes

4. When ready transfer to the mashed banana
    mixture and mix well

5. Serve when ready

Serves: *2*
Prep Time: *5*   Minutes

Cook Time: *10*   Minutes

Total Time: *15*   Minutes

INGREDIENTS

- 1 cup oats
- 2 cup almond milk
- 1 tablespoon maple syrup
- 1 banana
- 1 tsp vanilla extract
- ¼ tsp cinnamon
- 1 tablespoon chia seeds

DIRECTIONS

1. Place all ingredients into a saucepan and bring to a boil
2. Simmer for 5-6 minutes
3. When ready remove from heat

4. Transfer to a bowl, top with walnuts and serve

Serves: *1*

Prep Time: *10* Minutes

Cook Time: *10* Minutes

Total Time: *20* Minutes

INGREDIENTS

- ¼ cup gluten free oats
- ¼ cup water
- ¼ cup almond milk
- 1 banana
- 1 tablespoon brown sugar
- ¼ tsp vanilla extract
- ½ cup cherries
- ¼ cup almonds

DIRECTIONS

1. In a saucepan add oats, water, banana, milk and cook for 4-5 minutes

2. When ready remove from heat and add
    remaining ingredients

3. Mix well and serve

Serves: **2**

Prep Time: *10*   Minutes

Cook Time: *30*   Minutes

Total Time: *40*   Minutes

INGREDIENTS

- 1 tablespoon olive oil
- 1 onion
- 1 cup spinach
- 1 avocado
- 4 eggs
- 2 cups cheese
- ¼ tsp salt

DIRECTIONS

1. In a skillet sauté onion until soft
2. In a bowl beat the eggs with salt
3. Add remaining ingredients and mix well
4. Place the mixture into a prepare baking dish

5. Bake at 325 F for 25-30 minutes

6. When ready remove from the oven and serve

ASPARAGUS FRITATTA

Serves: **2**

Prep Time: **10**   Minutes

Cook Time: **20**   Minutes

Total Time: **30**   Minutes

INGREDIENTS

- ½ lb. asparagus
- 1 tablespoon olive oil
- ½ red onion
- ¼ tsp salt
- 2 oz. cheddar cheese
- 1 garlic clove
- ¼ tsp dill

DIRECTIONS

1. Boil the asparagus until tender and set aside
2. In a bowl whisk eggs with salt and cheese

3. In a frying pan heat olive oil and pour egg mixture

4. Add remaining ingredients and mix well

5. When ready serve with asparagus

SQUASH FRITATTA

Serves: **2**

Prep Time: **10**   Minutes

Cook Time: **20**   Minutes

Total Time: **30**   Minutes

INGREDIENTS

- ½ lb. squash
- 1 tablespoon olive oil
- ½ red onion
- ¼ tsp salt
- 2 oz. cheddar cheese
- 1 garlic clove
- ¼ tsp dill

DIRECTIONS

1. In a bowl whisk eggs with salt and cheese
2. In a frying pan heat olive oil and pour egg mixture
3. Add remaining ingredients and mix well

4. Serve when ready

Serves: *2*

Prep Time: *10*   Minutes

Cook Time: *20*   Minutes

Total Time: *30*   Minutes

INGREDIENTS

- 1 cup kale
- 1 tablespoon olive oil
- ½ red onion
- ¼ tsp salt
- 2 oz. cheddar cheese
- 1 garlic clove
- ¼ tsp dill

DIRECTIONS

1. In a skillet sauté kale until tender
2. In a bowl whisk eggs with salt and cheese
3. In a frying pan heat olive oil and pour egg mixture

4. Add remaining ingredients and mix well
5. When ready serve with sautéed kale

SPROUTS FRITATTA

Serves: **2**

Prep Time: **10**   Minutes

Cook Time: **20**   Minutes

Total Time: **30**   Minutes

INGREDIENTS

- ½ lb. sprouts
- 1 tablespoon olive oil
- ½ red onion
- ¼ tsp salt
- 2 oz. parmesan cheese
- 1 garlic clove
- ¼ tsp dill

DIRECTIONS

1. In a bowl whisk eggs with salt and parmesan cheese

2. In a frying pan heat olive oil and pour egg mixture

3. Add remaining ingredients and mix well
4. Serve when ready

BROCCOLI FRITATTA

Serves: **2**

Prep Time: **10**   Minutes

Cook Time: **20**   Minutes

Total Time: **30**   Minutes

INGREDIENTS

- 1 cup broccoli
- 1 tablespoon olive oil
- ½ red onion
- ¼ tsp salt
- 2 oz. cheddar cheese
- 1 garlic clove
- ¼ tsp dill

DIRECTIONS

1. In a skillet sauté broccoli until tender
2. In a bowl whisk eggs with salt and cheese
3. In a frying pan heat olive oil and pour egg mixture

4. Add remaining ingredients and mix well
5. When ready serve with sautéed broccoli

CAULIFLOWER STEAKS WITH LEMON SAUCE

57

Serves: **4**
Prep Time: **10**   Minutes

Cook Time: **10**   Minutes

Total Time: **20**   Minutes

INGREDIENTS

- 1 head cauliflower
- 2 tablespoons olive oil
- 2 tsp paprika

LEMON SAUCE

- 1 cup parsley leaves
- ¼ cup mint leaves
- 1 garlic clove
- ¼ cup olive oil
- ¼ cup green onion
- Juice of 1 lemon

DIRECTIONS

1. In a blender add all ingredients for the lemon sauce and blend until smooth

2. For the cauliflower steak, cut cauliflower into thick slices and rub with olive oil

3. Sprinkle with spices and place the cauliflower in a skillet

4. Cook for 4-5 minutes per side

5. When ready remove and serve with lemon sauce

RICE, KALE AND AVOCADO BOWL

Serves: **2**

Prep Time: **10**   Minutes

Cook Time: **20**   Minutes

Total Time: **30**   Minutes

INGREDIENTS

- 1 cup rice
- 1 garlic clove
- 1 tablespoon rice vinegar
- 2 cups vegetable broth
- pinch of salt
- pinch of pepper
- 2 tablespoons
- 1 bunch kale
- 1 bunch kale
- 1 avocado

DIRECTIONS

1. In a pot stir in broth, rice and garlic

2. Bring to a simmer for and cook until liquid is evaporated

3. When ready toss rice with salt, pepper and vinegar

4. In another books toss kale with olive oil

5. Add kale and avocado slices to the rice

6. Serve when ready

CHICKEN MEATBALLS AND CAULIFLOWER RICE

Serves:	*4*
Prep Time:	*10* Minutes
Cook Time:	*30* Minutes
Total Time:	*40* Minutes

INGREDIENTS

- ¼ cup red onion
- 1 lb. ground chicken
- 1 tablespoon mustard
- ¼ tsp black pepper
- 1 tablespoon olive oil
- 1 garlic clove
- ¼ cup parsley
- pinch of salt

SAUCE

- 1 cup parsley
- 1 can coconut milk
- 2 scallions

- zest of 1 lemon
- 1 cup ready-made cauliflower rice

DIRECTIONS

1. In a skillet heat olive oil and sauté onion and garlic for 3-4 minutes
2. Remove sautéed onion and garlic to a bowl
3. Stir in parsley, mustard, chicken, seasoning and mix well
4. Form balls from the mixture and place on a baking sheet
5. Bake at 400 F for 20 minutes
6. When ready remove from the oven and set aside
7. In a blender add all ingredients for the sauce and blend
8. Top the meatballs with sauce and cauliflower rice and serve

Serves: **2**
Prep Time: **10**   Minutes

Cook Time: **15**   Minutes

Total Time: **25**   Minutes

INGREDIENTS

- **1 cup red bell pepper**
- **¼ cup cucumber**
- **¼ cup zucchini**
- **¼ cup asparagus**
- **¼ cup carrots**
- **1 onion**
- **2 eggs**
- **1 tsp salt**
- **1 tsp pepper**
- **Seasoning**
- **1 tablespoon olive oil**

DIRECTIONS

1. In a skillet heat olive oil and sauté onion until soft

2. Chop vegetables into thin slices and pour over onion

3. Whisk eggs with salt and pepper and pour over the vegetables

4. Cook until vegetables are brown

5. When ready remove from heat and serve

Serves: *4*

Prep Time: *10*   Minutes

Cook Time: *55*   Minutes

Total Time: *65*   Minutes

INGREDIENTS

- 1 onion
- 2 garlic cloves
- ¼ lb. carrots
- 1 potato
- 1 tablespoon balsamic vinegar
- ¼ tsp salt
- ¼ tsp black pepper
- 1 tablespoon olive oil
- 1 cup water

DIRECTIONS

1. **Chop all the vegetables and place them in a heated skillet**

2. Add remaining ingredients and cook on low heat

3. Allow to simmer for 40-45 minutes or until
    vegetables are soft

4. Transfer mixture to a blender and blend until
    smooth

5. When ready remove from the blender and serve

BRUSSELS SPROUT SALAD

Serves: 2
Prep Time: 5   Minutes

Cook Time: 5   Minutes

Total Time: *10*   Minutes

INGREDIENTS

- 1 tablespoon olive oil
- 1 cup shallots
- ½ cup celery
- 1 clove garlic
- 6-8 brussels sprouts
- 1 tablespoon thyme leaves
- herbs

DIRECTIONS

1. In a bowl mix all ingredients and mix well
2. Serve with dressing

Serves: **2**

Prep Time: **5**   Minutes

Cook Time: **5**   Minutes

Total Time: ***10***   Minutes

INGREDIENTS

- ¼ cup almonds
- 4 oz. goat cheese
- 4 cups salad greens
- 1 tablespoon olive oil
- 2-3 pears
- 2 tablespoons honey

DIRECTIONS

1. In a bowl mix all ingredients and mix well
2. Serve with dressing

GREEN SALAD

Serves: *2*

Prep Time: *5*   Minutes

Cook Time: *5*   Minutes

Total Time: *10*   Minutes

INGREDIENTS

- 2 garlic cloves
- 1 tsp mustard
- 1 bunch watercress
- 2 oz. rocket leaves
- ½ lb. tomatoes
- ½ cup radishes
- 2 tablespoons olive oil

DIRECTIONS

1. In a bowl mix all ingredients and mix well
2. Serve with dressing

Serves: **2**
Prep Time: **5**   Minutes

Cook Time: **5**   Minutes

Total Time: **10**   Minutes

INGREDIENTS

- 1 garlic clove
- 1 tablespoon red wine vinegar
- 4 tomatoes
- 8 cherry tomatoes
- 4 radishes
- 4 radicchio leaves
- ½ cup basil leaves

DIRECTIONS

1. In a bowl mix all ingredients and mix well
2. Serve with dressing

FENNEL & FETA SALAD

Serves: **2**
Prep Time: **5**   Minutes

Cook Time: **5**   Minutes

Total Time: *10*   Minutes

INGREDIENTS

- 2 fennel bulbs
- ¼ lb. peas
- 1 bunch mint
- ¼ lb. yogurt
- 1 tablespoon olive oil
- ½ cup feta cheese

DIRECTIONS

1. In a bowl mix all ingredients and mix well
2. Serve with dressing

Serves: **2**

Prep Time: **5**   Minutes

Cook Time: **5**   Minutes

Total Time: **10**   Minutes

INGREDIENTS

- ½ lb. egg noodles
- 1 tsp chili flakes
- 1 tsp sesame oil
- 1 tablespoon honey
- 1 lb. cooked turkey
- 1 avocado
- 1 bunch coriander
- ½ cucumber
- ½ lb. tomatoes

DIRECTIONS

1. In a bowl mix all ingredients and mix well
2. Serve with dressing

RAINBOW SALAD

73

Serves: **2**

Prep Time: **5**   Minutes

Cook Time: **5**   Minutes

Total Time: **10**   Minutes

INGREDIENTS

- 1 lb. green beans
- 2 bunch rainbow carrots
- 1 bunch radishes
- 1 red onion
- ½ lb. baby leaf salad mix
- 2 tablespoons olive oil
- 1 tsp salt
- ½ cup cashews

DIRECTIONS

1. In a bowl mix all ingredients and mix well
3. Serve with dressing

Serves: **2**

Prep Time: **5**   Minutes

Cook Time: **5**   Minutes

Total Time: ***10***   Minutes

INGREDIENTS

- 2 cloves garlic
- 2 onions
- 1 green chili
- 8 grilled banana prawns
- 1 lemon
- 2 tomatoes
- 1 avocado

DIRECTIONS

1. In a bowl mix all ingredients and mix well
4. Serve with dressing

BLACK BEAN SALAD

Serves:　　　　**2**

Prep Time:　　**5**　Minutes

Cook Time:　　**5**　Minutes

Total Time:　**10**　Minutes

INGREDIENTS

- 1 cup corn
- 2 tablespoons olive oil
- 2 oz. jalapeno chilies
- ¼ lb. sour cream
- 1 can black beans
- 2 tomatoes
- 1 red onion
- 1 avocado

DIRECTIONS

1. In a bowl mix all ingredients and mix well
2. Serve with dressing

Serves: **2**
Prep Time: **5** Minutes

Cook Time: **5** Minutes

Total Time: **10** Minutes

INGREDIENTS

- 1 cup bread crumbs
- ½ lb. goat cheese
- 1 egg
- 1 avocado
- 2 oz watercress
- 8 baby greens
- 1 tomato

DIRECTIONS

1. In a bowl mix all ingredients and mix well
2. Serve with dressing

SIMPLE PIZZA RECIPE

Serves: **6-8**
Prep Time: **10**   Minutes

Cook Time: **15**   Minutes

Total Time: **25**   Minutes

INGREDIENTS

- 1 pizza crust
- ½ cup tomato sauce
- ¼ black pepper
- 1 cup pepperoni slices
- 1 cup mozzarella cheese
- 1 cup olives

DIRECTIONS

1. Spread tomato sauce on the pizza crust
2. Place all the toppings on the pizza crust
3. Bake the pizza at 425 F for 12-15 minutes

4. When ready remove pizza from the oven and
    serve

79

Serves: *6-8*
Prep Time: *10*   Minutes

Cook Time: *15*   Minutes

Total Time: *25*   Minutes

INGREDIENTS

- 1 pizza crust
- ½ cup tomato sauce
- ¼ black pepper
- 1 cup zucchini slices
- 1 cup mozzarella cheese
- 1 cup olives

DIRECTIONS

1. Spread tomato sauce on the pizza crust
2. Place all the toppings on the pizza crust
3. Bake the pizza at 425 F for 12-15 minutes
4. When ready remove pizza from the oven and serve

CAULIFLOWER RECIPE

Serves: **6-8**

Prep Time: **10**   Minutes

Cook Time: **15**   Minutes

Total Time: **25**   Minutes

INGREDIENTS

- 1 pizza crust
- ½ cup tomato sauce
- ¼ black pepper
- 1 cup cauliflower
- 1 cup mozzarella cheese
- 1 cup olives

DIRECTIONS

1. Spread tomato sauce on the pizza crust
2. Place all the toppings on the pizza crust
3. Bake the pizza at 425 F for 12-15 minutes
4. When ready remove pizza from the oven and serve

Serves:	*6-8*
Prep Time:	*10* Minutes
Cook Time:	*15* Minutes
Total Time:	*25* Minutes

INGREDIENTS

- 1 pizza crust
- ½ cup tomato sauce
- ¼ black pepper
- 1 cup broccoli
- 1 cup mozzarella cheese
- 1 cup olives

DIRECTIONS

1. Spread tomato sauce on the pizza crust
2. Place all the toppings on the pizza crust
3. Bake the pizza at 425 F for 12-15 minutes
4. When ready remove pizza from the oven and serve

TOMATOES & HAM PIZZA

Serves: *6-8*
Prep Time: *10*   Minutes

Cook Time: *15*   Minutes

Total Time: *25*   Minutes

INGREDIENTS

- 1 pizza crust
- ½ cup tomato sauce
- ¼ black pepper
- 1 cup pepperoni slices
- 1 cup tomatoes
- 6-8 ham slices
- 1 cup mozzarella cheese
- 1 cup olives

DIRECTIONS

1. Spread tomato sauce on the pizza crust
2. Place all the toppings on the pizza crust
3. Bake the pizza at 425 F for 12-15 minutes

4. When ready remove pizza from the oven and
    serve

84

Serves:	**4**
Prep Time:	**10** Minutes
Cook Time:	**20** Minutes
Total Time:	**30** Minutes

INGREDIENTS

- 1 tablespoon olive oil
- 1 lb. turnip
- ¼ red onion
- ½ cup all-purpose flour
- ¼ tsp salt
- ¼ tsp pepper
- 1 can vegetable broth
- 1 cup heavy cream

DIRECTIONS

1. In a saucepan heat olive oil and sauté onion until tender

2. Add remaining ingredients to the saucepan and bring to a boil

3. When all the vegetables are tender transfer to a blender and blend until smooth

4. Pour soup into bowls, garnish with parsley and serve

ZUCCHINI SOUP

Serves:	*4*
Prep Time:	*10* Minutes
Cook Time:	*20* Minutes
Total Time:	*30* Minutes

INGREDIENTS

- 1 tablespoon olive oil
- 1 lb. zucchini
- ¼ red onion
- ½ cup all-purpose flour
- ¼ tsp salt
- ¼ tsp pepper
- 1 can vegetable broth
- 1 cup heavy cream

DIRECTIONS

1. **In a saucepan heat olive oil and sauté zucchini until tender**

2. Add remaining ingredients to the saucepan and bring to a boil

3. When all the vegetables are tender transfer to a blender and blend until smooth

4. Pour soup into bowls, garnish with parsley and serve

Serves: **4**

Prep Time: **10** Minutes

Cook Time: **20** Minutes

Total Time: **30** Minutes

INGREDIENTS

- 1 tablespoon olive oil
- 1 lb. watercress
- ¼ red onion
- ½ cup all-purpose flour
- ¼ tsp salt
- ¼ tsp pepper
- 1 can vegetable broth
- 1 cup heavy cream

DIRECTIONS

1. **In a saucepan heat olive oil and sauté onion until tender**

2. Add remaining ingredients to the saucepan and bring to a boil

3. When all the vegetables are tender transfer to a blender and blend until smooth

4. Pour soup into bowls, garnish with parsley and serve

CARROT SOUP

Serves: *4*

Prep Time: *10*   Minutes

Cook Time: *20*   Minutes

Total Time: *30*   Minutes

INGREDIENTS

- 1 tablespoon olive oil
- 1 lb. carrots
- ¼ red onion
- ½ cup all-purpose flour
- ¼ tsp salt
- ¼ tsp pepper
- 1 can vegetable broth
- 1 cup heavy cream

DIRECTIONS

1. **In a saucepan heat olive oil and sauté carrots until tender**

2. Add remaining ingredients to the saucepan and bring to a boil

3. When all the vegetables are tender transfer to a blender and blend until smooth

4. Pour soup into bowls, garnish with parsley and serve

Serves: *4*
Prep Time: *10*   Minutes

Cook Time: *20*   Minutes

Total Time: *30*   Minutes

INGREDIENTS

- 1 tablespoon olive oil
- 1 lb. black beans
- ¼ red onion
- ½ cup all-purpose flour
- ¼ tsp salt
- ¼ tsp pepper
- 1 can vegetable broth
- 1 cup heavy cream

DIRECTIONS

1. **In a saucepan heat olive oil and sauté onion until tender**

2. Add remaining ingredients to the saucepan and bring to a boil

3. When all the vegetables are tender transfer to a blender and blend until smooth

4. Pour soup into bowls, garnish with parsley and serve

POMEGRANATE SMOOTHIE

Serves: *1*
Prep Time: *5*   Minutes

Cook Time: *5*   Minutes

Total Time: *10* Minutes

INGREDIENTS

- 1 banana
- 1 cup pomegranate juice
- 1 cup Greek yogurt
- 1 cup ice

DIRECTIONS

1. In a blender place all ingredients and blend until smooth
2. Pour smoothie in a glass and serve

Serves: *1*
Prep Time: *5*   Minutes

Cook Time: *5*   Minutes

Total Time: *10*   Minutes

INGREDIENTS

- 1 cup pineapple
- 1 banana
- 1 orange
- 1 cup

DIRECTIONS

1. In a blender place all ingredients and blend until smooth
2. Pour smoothie in a glass and serve

Serves: *1*
Prep Time: **5**   Minutes

Cook Time: **5**   Minutes

Total Time: *10*   Minutes

INGREDIENTS

- 2 tablespoons pumpkin
- 4 tablespoons coconut milk
- 1 tsp honey
- 1 banana
- ¼ tsp cinnamon
- 1 cup ice

DIRECTIONS

1. In a blender place all ingredients and blend until smooth
2. Pour smoothie in a glass and serve

KIWI SMOOTHIE

Serves: *1*

Prep Time: *5*   Minutes

Cook Time: *5*   Minutes

Total Time: *10* Minutes

INGREDIENTS

- 2 kiwis
- 2 bananas
- 1 cup soy milk
- 1 cup yogurt
- 2 tablespoons porridge oats
- 1 tsp honey

DIRECTIONS

1. In a blender place all ingredients and blend until smooth
2. Pour smoothie in a glass and serve

BERRY KALE SMOOTHIE

Serves: *1*
Prep Time: *5*   Minutes

Cook Time: *5*   Minutes

Total Time: *10*   Minutes

INGREDIENTS

- 1 handful kale
- 1 banana
- 1 cup berries
- 1 cup almond milk
- 1 cup protein powder

DIRECTIONS

1. In a blender place all ingredients and blend until smooth
2. Pour smoothie in a glass and serve

COCONUT SMOOTHIE

Serves: *1*
Prep Time: *5*   Minutes

Cook Time: *5*   Minutes

Total Time: *10*   Minutes

INGREDIENTS

- 1 cup coconut milk
- ½ cup pineapple chunks
- 1 banana
- ½ cup pineapple juice
- 1 cup ice

DIRECTIONS

1. In a blender place all ingredients and blend until smooth
2. Pour smoothie in a glass and serve

AVOCADO SMOOTHIE

Serves: *1*

Prep Time: **5**   Minutes

Cook Time: **5**   Minutes

Total Time: **10**   Minutes

INGREDIENTS

- 1 cup coconut milk
- 1 cup pineapple chunks
- 1 avocado
- 1 banana
- 1 tsp vanilla extract
- 1 tablespoon hemp seeds
- 1 cup ice

DIRECTIONS

1. In a blender place all ingredients and blend until smooth
2. Pour smoothie in a glass and serve

TURMERIC SMOOTHIE

Serves: *1*
Prep Time: *5*   Minutes

Cook Time: *5*   Minutes

Total Time: *10* Minutes

INGREDIENTS

- 1 banana
- 1 cup almond milk
- 1 tsp turmeric
- 1 tsp ginger
- 1 tsp cinnamon
- 1 tsp honey
- 1 cup ice

DIRECTIONS

1. In a blender place all ingredients and blend until smooth
2. Pour smoothie in a glass and serve

PAPAYA SMOOTHIE

Serves: *1*
Prep Time: 5   Minutes

Cook Time: 5   Minutes

Total Time: *10* Minutes

INGREDIENTS

- 1 banana
- 1 cup papaya
- 1 cup blueberries
- 1 tsp cinnamon
- 1 cup spinach
- 1 tablespoon chia seeds
- 1 cup almond milk

DIRECTIONS

1. **In a blender place all ingredients and blend until smooth**
2. **Pour smoothie in a glass and serve**

Serves: *1*

Prep Time: 5 Minutes

Cook Time: 5 Minutes

Total Time: *10* Minutes

INGREDIENTS

- 1 apple
- 1 cup spinach
- 1 cup kale
- 1 cup ice

DIRECTIONS

1. **In a blender place all ingredients and blend until smooth**
2. **Pour smoothie in a glass and serve**

THANK YOU FOR READING THIS BOOK!

www.ingramcontent.com/pod-product-compliance
Lightning Source LLC
Chambersburg PA
CBHW031255250726
48655CB00005B/2233